CW01011471

Contents

Introduction

Aims of this guide

This guide provides an overview of the evidence that group singing can be beneficial for respiratory health and wellbeing. It also gives information and guidance on setting up singing groups for people living in the community who have experience of diagnosed COPD. This includes conditions such as bronchitis and emphysema. Such singing groups may also seek to involve family, friends and carers of people with COPD.

The guide draws upon the experience of COPD patients in a number of well-established community singing for COPD groups as well as musicians with considerable experience of running such groups. It draws especially upon the experience of musicians and health researchers in the Sidney De Haan Research Centre for Arts and Health in establishing and evaluating a network of singing groups for COPD patients and their supporters, which began in September 2009.

Who is this guide for?

This guide is for anyone interested in setting up, running and evaluating singing groups for the benefit of people with COPD living in the community. This includes:

- Health professionals, such as specialist respiratory nurses or physiotherapists involved in pulmonary rehabilitation who want to develop evidence-based community activities to promote the wellbeing of people with COPD

- Voluntary sector organisations and support groups, such as British Lung Foundation Breathe Easy Groups who would like to set up singing groups for people with COPD

- People experiencing COPD, whether mild, moderate, severe, or very severe, who are attempting to self-manage their condition

- Family, relatives and friends of people with COPD who are looking for an effective means of engagement and social support for their loved ones

- Experienced community musicians interested in setting up singing for health groups who have not previously worked with people with COPD

What this guide offers

Information is provided on evidence from case studies and research projects, and links to further resources and training. This is not intended as a practical toolkit, but to guide and inform.

Context

The nature and scale of COPD in the UK

COPD is an umbrella term for a number of specific conditions leading to irreversible airflow obstruction including bronchitis and emphysema.

Diagnosis relies on a combination of history, physical examination and confirmation of airflow obstruction using spirometry (NIHCE, 2010). Four stages of COPD severity can be distinguished – mild, moderate, severe and very severe (GOLD, 2009). Severe COPD is indicated by an FEV_1 of <50% and >30% of expected values for age and sex, and very severe indicated by an FEV_1 value of <30%.

> Forced expiratory volume (FEV_1) is the volume of air exhaled in one second when the patient inhales maximally and then exhales as forcefully and deeply as possible (Halpin, 2003:26).

The most common debilitating symptom of COPD is breathlessness (Thorax, 2004), which often leads to inactivity, isolation and dependence. Pulmonary Rehabilitation can improve physical activity and quality of life, although the benefits depend upon continued adherence to physical activity (BTS/BLF, 2002). COPD is associated with other, often smoking-related long-term health conditions including cardiovascular disease, osteoporosis and depression (Fletcher, van der Molen, Salapatas et al., 2010). As Jones notes (Jones, 2009) COPD is characterised by 'a spiral of decline': 'As COPD progresses, patients fail to exercise, feel depressed, and experience low self-esteem.'

In England, approximately 835,000 people have been diagnosed with COPD, but the true prevalence is likely to be over 3 million (DH, 2010a). In an average UK health district of 250,000 people, GPs will have 14,200 consultations a year from patients with COPD and 680 patients will be admitted to hospital (BTS/BLF 2002).

Exacerbation of COPD is the second most common cause of emergency admissions to hospitals in the UK and one of the most expensive conditions treated by the NHS (BLF, 2007) with direct costs of £810 – £930 million per year, which are expected to rise (DH, 2010a). COPD mainly affects people beyond retirement age, but 24 million lost working days a year are due to COPD (BTS/BLF, 2002). The Department of Health consultation on a strategy for COPD in England (DH, 2010a) highlighted the need to improve prevention efforts, support early identification, ensure accurate diagnosis and ensure high quality care of people with the disease and at the end of life. The strategy 'lays great emphasis on local health and social care and the third sector taking responsibility for contributing to service change and improvement.'

The Department of Health published a new cross-government strategy for COPD in July 2011 – 'National strategy to transform respiratory disease care'. This new strategy is intended to transform the care, quality of life and health outcomes for people with COPD and will drive improvements in outcomes for patients.

Pharmaceuticals

Treatment of COPD depends upon what symptoms are present and the extent of the lung damage. Some patients only need a course of antibiotics following an exacerbation. Patients with regular symptoms may use an inhaler, and advanced cases may be given oxygen to breathe. Steroids are used for some patients following an exacerbation, and a few patients are prescribed regular steroid tablets (Halpin, 2003, p66).

There is a well-known deterioration curve, so the best that can be hoped for physically is maintenance of lung function, i.e. attempting to slow down the deterioration, and to 'manage' breathing by relaxed breathing control techniques. Psychologically, improved confidence by using breathing techniques will improve perceived wellbeing, and help to reduce isolation. Wellbeing can be further improved by providing a safe, friendly singing group environment, where supportive friendships can form, and social inclusion can be fostered through performances.

Living in the community

Patients living in the community may be supported by their GP who may have a Nurse Respiratory Specialist in the practice, and may have been referred to the Pulmonary Rehabilitation Team for a course of rehabilitation. The British Lung Foundation (BLF) has a network of 'Breathe Easy' Groups in the community, which provide support to patients. Referrals to a singing for breathing group could come from these supporters, and GPs, Nurse Respiratory Specialists, the Pulmonary Rehabilitation Team, and BLF Nurses. They could also provide group organisers and facilitators with support in any cases of any difficulties or relapse of the participant. Referral is discussed in detail in a separate section below.

Social support in recovery

The medical Model consists of diagnosis, treatment and cure, or management of the condition if cure isn't possible. A patient supported by the clinical staff and at a stage in their condition that they are able to live in the community, possibly with the support of third sector voluntary organisations, may be ready to engage activities that can help them improve their sense of wellbeing and quality of life, and re-engagement with others.

Here, the emphasis is on supporting patients' social needs and their gradually increasing empowerment in choice and directing their lives, which includes education, employment, income, housing etc.

From this point of view, ill health can be seen as period of profound loss for the patient of the following features of good psychological and social health wellbeing:

- Positive feelings
- Self-belief
- Social support and network
- Expectation and hope
- Abilities and skills
- Organisation and structure

People with chronic health challenges need support and interventions to help them re-build or develop these aspects of wellbeing. People who actively engage in group singing can benefit in these many different ways.

The salutogenic model of health

A useful model of positive health comes from the perspective of Health Promotion and Antonovsky's salutogenic model of health (Antonovsky, 1987 and 1996). In Antonovsky's model, good health is promoted through 'generalised resistance resources'. It is when resistance resources are inadequate to restore health balance, or manage stress, that an individual breaks down (Antonovsky, 1972). These resistance resources are represented by the concept of 'sense of coherence', which consists of three components: comprehensibility, manageability and meaningfulness (Antonovsky, 1987 and 1993), and these are defined as follows:

Sense of coherence: A global orientation that expresses the extent to which one has a pervasive, enduring though dynamic feeling of confidence that:

- the stimuli deriving from one's internal and external environments in the course of living are structured, predictable, and explicable; .
- the resources are available to one to meet the demands posed by the stimuli;
- these demands are challenges, worthy of investment and engagement.

Antonovsky (1987, p19)

Comprehensibility: The person who experiences the world as comprehensible expects that future stimuli will be predictable or, when they do come as surprises, will be orderable and explicable.

Manageability: People who experience their world as manageable have the sense that, aided by their own resources or by those of trustworthy others, they will be able to cope.

Meaningfulness: A person who experiences the world as meaningful will not be overcome by unhappy experiences but will experience them as challenges, be determined to seek meaning in them, and do his/her best to overcome them with dignity.

Carstens and Spangenberg (1997, p1212)

For a recent review of Salutogenesis, see Lindstrom and Eriksson, 2010.

Personal experiences of COPD

Personal narratives from people affected by COPD are also invaluable in understanding how COPD can develop and the effects it has on people's lives. Jean Fraser is an artist living in Whitstable and an associate of the Sidney De Haan Research Centre for Arts and Health and key member of the team developing our work on singing and COPD. Jean describes herself as a 'health activist' and has demonstrated through her artistic project 'Breathing Space' in which she undertook a coastal cycle journey around the coast of Kent promoting awareness of COPD, that a physically active life is still possible despite obstructed lung function. It exemplifies the Salutogenic approach of providing meaningfulness (motivation, purpose), comprehensibility (understanding), and manageability (have the resources, or can obtain them).

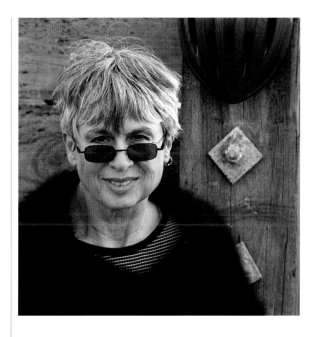

Jean Fraser talks about living with COPD

"I am a photographic artist, mother, lover, environmental and health activist, retired NHS art therapist. I am also a person living with (rather than suffering from) severe COPD, an active member of my local Breathe Easy group, and an Expert Patients Programme tutor. Diagnosed in 2000, aged fifty four, I looked up the root of diagnosis, discovering that the Greek compound dia means 'apart/split', and gnosi 'knowledge'; or put another way, split apart by knowledge. And split apart was how I felt when, terrified; I fled my London home for the healthier air of the Kent coast.

My understanding of COPD had been that it was a death sentence. I was deeply shocked as I had assumed that my cigarette consumption (10 packs a year) was insufficient risk for the dreaded emphysema I had heard about from my parents. I was ignorant of genetic and environmental co-factors – chemicals from my photographic darkroom practice, dust from frequent bouts of house-building during which I seldom wore a mask.

As I had understood it, newly diagnosed patients were told to go home and rest, a euphemism for waiting to die. As a moderate smoker who quit aged 40, imminent mortality didn't seem fair. At this point all I knew about COPD was that it progressively deprives you of oxygen. What I couldn't yet envisage was that the disease's challenge, in conjunction with excellent clinical care from my consultant, the local specialist respiratory team and my GP, would set me on a new path which would give my life new meaning." Based on: Fraser, Page and Skingley (2011)

The current national policy framework for COPD

The Department of Health published a new cross-government strategy for COPD in July 2011 – 'National strategy to transform respiratory disease care'. This new strategy is intended to transform the care, quality of life and health outcomes for people with COPD and will drive improvements in outcomes for patients. Coordinating the efforts of the NHS, patients, social care and voluntary organisations, the strategy aims to help people avoid lung disease and to promote longer and healthier lives for those with the condition, through coordinating the efforts of the NHS, and social care and voluntary organisations, and through promoting more effective self-management strategies on the part of patients themselves. The strategy will promote:

- Respiratory health and good lung health
- Early accurate diagnosis
- Active partnership between healthcare professionals and people with COPD/asthma
- Chronic disease management (and good control of symptoms)
- Targeted evidence-based treatment for the individual

Everyone affected by COPD and asthma can also expect to have a care planning discussion with their healthcare professional. This will allow individuals to personalise their care and plan their lung health on an ongoing basis so that they can identify any problems and seek help before their symptoms worsen.

The Outcomes Strategy identifies six objectives that will drive work to transform respiratory care within the health and social care system:

- Better prevention of COPD
- Reducing premature death
- Improving quality of life
- Improving safe and effective care
- Reducing the impact of asthma
- Reducing inequalities in access to and quality of services

While the NHS has a key role in achieving these objectives, it cannot do so alone, and effective partnerships between pulmonary rehabilitation services, community respiratory nurses, respiratory nurses in GP practices, British Lung Foundation nurses, local government and charitable and voluntary organisations, are key. The argument of this guide is that community opportunities for people to come together and sing could make a considerable contribution to achieving these objectives – as could many other forms of creative activity and cultural participation. However, singing can be undertaken by almost everybody, even sitting down; all that is needed is to be able to speak, and hear (to be tuneful).

When people with a history of COPD come together to sing guided by a sensitive and skilled facilitator, they are taking part in an activity, which is inherently caring and supportive. Members of choirs get to know one another, form friendships and offer support for one another. For these reasons alone, the experience can contribute to the process of rehabilitation, but in addition there are inherent features of singing and learning new material, which helps to promote a sense of wellbeing. Not least is the enjoyment and fun associated with singing; the concentration and sense of achievement that comes from learning something new; the sense of working together in a team cooperatively, and finally the beauty of the final result in performance.

Singing together reflects in fact, all five of the Five Ways to Wellbeing devised by the New Economics Foundation Wellbeing Programme:

- Connect – with people around you
- Be active – walk, run, cycle, dance
- Take notice – catch sight of the beautiful, savour the moment
- Keep learning – makes you more confident as well as being fun
- Give – do something nice for a friend or a stranger

How group singing can help promote wellbeing and quality of life for people with COPD

Group singing can help to address all of the social needs identified above of patients living in the community, with support, and ready to engage socially.

Positive feelings: Singing has been shown to be a joyful and uplifting experience. It generates a sense of positive mood, happiness and enjoyment. Such positive feelings also counteract feelings of stress or anxiety and help to distract people from internal negative thoughts and feelings.

Expectation and hope: Enjoyable activities such as singing with others are things people will look forward to each week. They can become highlights of the week and positive memories remain alive for hours and days afterwards. Where an activity involves working towards a goal such as a performance, there are enhanced expectations of rewarding outcomes.

Self-belief: A change of identity can occur for people with COPD by participating in group singing, from thinking of themselves as choir members, rather than patients. This can raise a sense of self-esteem and confidence and performance events can bring a sense of social recognition and status. Performances help to reduce stigma and labelling by others.

Abilities and skills: Confidence is brought about by the ability to repeat previously learned tasks or skills (including social skills), with a high degree of accuracy. Successful skills might also help to improve success in new, related skills, when tried for the first time. Learning new songs or harmonising parts of songs, can help concentration and focus, and stimulate learning and memory. Concentration can also provide a distraction from other concerns, leading to respite from them.

Social support and networking: Singing in a group offers the opportunity to build social capital, encourage social inclusion and raised status of the members, and creates an opportunity for communities to come together.

Organisation and structure: Structure is something that is easily lost when ill. Patients can feel adrift and disconnected. Having the purpose and goal of attending a weekly group, can be motivating and create an anchor upon which other weekly activities might build.

Evidence

Case studies

Case studies provide the most abundant evidence of the value of group singing for wellbeing. Across the UK, a few community singing groups have been established for people affected by the challenges of COPD. Two are known in Sussex, one on Brighton and one in Hove, which have been running for around four years, and one in Folkestone for two years. These groups have proved their value in practice. People with COPD would not continue attending singing groups if they didn't derive substantial benefits from the experience. We give here short case studies of these singing groups. In addition, the Royal Brompton and Harefield Hospital in London has run 'Singing for Breathing' groups for over two years as part of an on-going research project to evaluate the benefits of singing for people with very severe COPD. We also include here an account from Jane Petto, a singer who has had half her lung removed and is also living with COPD.

BetterBreathing singing groups (Brighton and Hove)

These singing groups were established in 2007 for people with breathing difficulties including COPD with funding from Brighton and Hove Primary Care Trust (PCT). The groups meet weekly and are led by musician and singing teacher Udita Everett with the support of an accompanist.

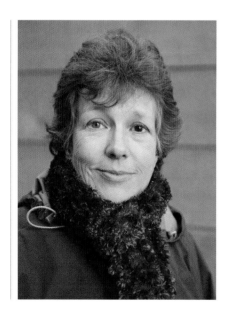

"The group is a lifeline to many local people. Members say that their health is greatly improved and it gives people a vital chance to make friends and meet others with the same difficulties. We always have a lot of fun!"

Udita Everitt
Leader, Brighton and Hove groups

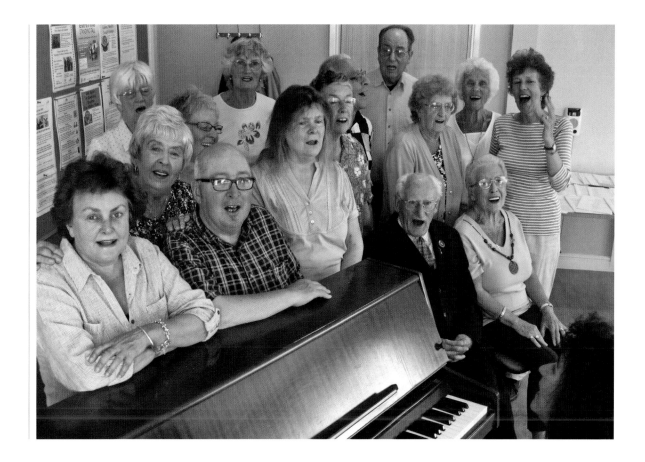

The project was the subject of a qualitative evaluation by a researcher for Brighton and Hove PCT, and positive feedback was gathered from members of the groups. They reported significant improvements to their health and wellbeing, including needing less medication, fewer trips to hospital, sleeping better and feeling less isolated. The following testimonials were given by group members:

"This group has been extremely helpful in many ways, physically and psychologically. I just don't have to worry about breathing any more. I am much calmer now and my sleep has improved."

"I am enjoying it very much, and I am improving my breathing and posture, and gaining more confidence!"

"My breathing has been maintained due to the exercise of singing and breathing, and it's kept me out of a hospital bed under the NHS. It has also helped me to give up cigarettes."

"The atmosphere is always welcoming, friendly and relaxed. New members are always made to feel at home. Afternoons fly by and you leave feeling uplifted and breathing easier."

"I go to the group with a tight chest, and leave feeling I can breathe again. The nurse measured my lung capacity: it improved through the singing classes!"

"The combination of relaxation, breathing exercises and singing is very therapeutic. I look forward to Mondays – sets me up for the week."

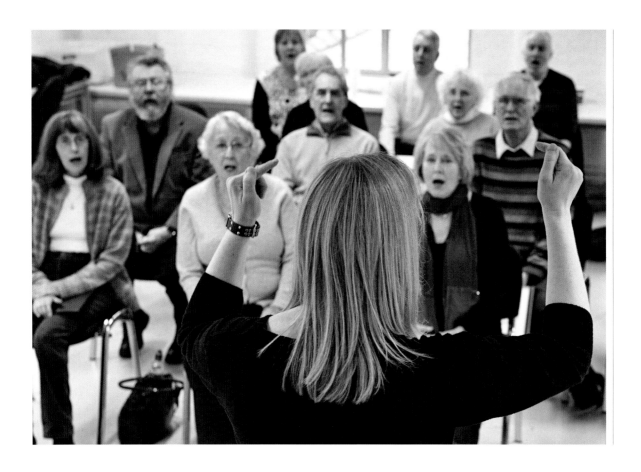

Singing for Breathing group (Folkestone)

The Folkestone Singing for Breathing group was set up by the Sidney De Haan Research Centre for Arts and Health as a pilot to help with the development of a more ambitious research project (see: Breathing Space, 2010). Each week, the members gather to sing simple rounds, songs and, most importantly, learn how to manage their breathing while singing. They are lead by Sonia Page, a respiratory specialist nurse and community musician. With practice week by week, the sound quality produced by the group has improved and Sonia has received positive feedback from the participants.

"Participants have told me that the group is helping them in very real terms: just feeling better, not having such a problem with sleep apnoea, which I've been surprised about, and feeling happier. I have absolute confidence in it helping, and I very much hope the end result is that people get this on prescription."

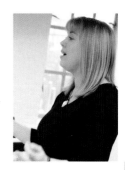

Sonia Page
Leader, 'Singing for Breathing' group, Folkestone

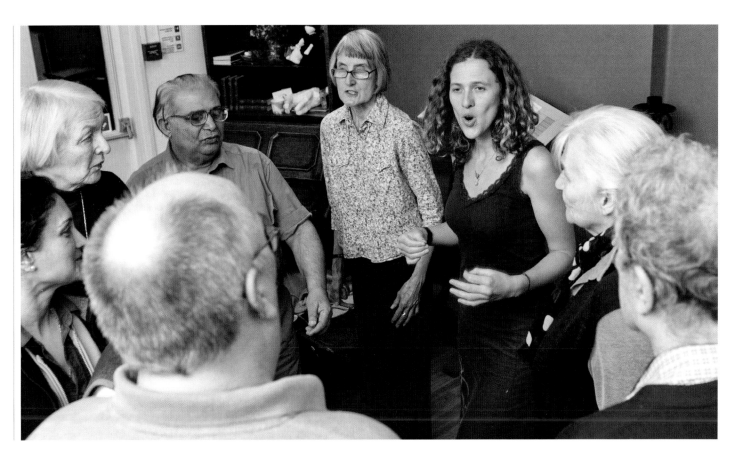

Singing for Breathing group, The Royal Brompton and Harefield Hospital (London)

For over four years singing groups have been running at the Royal Brompton and Harefield Hospital in London for in-patients and out-patients with severe COPD. The project is managed by Vicki Hume, director of the arts programme in the hospital and groups have been facilitated by Phoene Cave and Maya Waldman. These singing groups have been part of an innovative controlled trial to assess the impact of singing on lung function but also on their mental and social wellbeing.

Qualitative evaluation of the group has shown that the sessions are enjoyable and patients feel that singing has benefited their breathing.

"It was excellent – although aware of how to breathe correctly – very rarely put into practise when having breathing difficulties – during this workshop – opportunity to breathe naturally – and put all of this into practise – in a fun way – well-facilitated – fun, interesting and helpful!"

"Explained about breathing properly – e.g. diaphragm breathing."

"Apprehensive at first, but more confident as it went along. Relaxing."

"Brilliant. Brought strangers together working as a group, making new friends, you do not feel awkward and had fun. Helped with breathing and beneficial."

"I think they are great fun and certainly help to break up a tedious hospital appointment. If they were to be a regular thing it would be something to look forward to every 3 weeks."

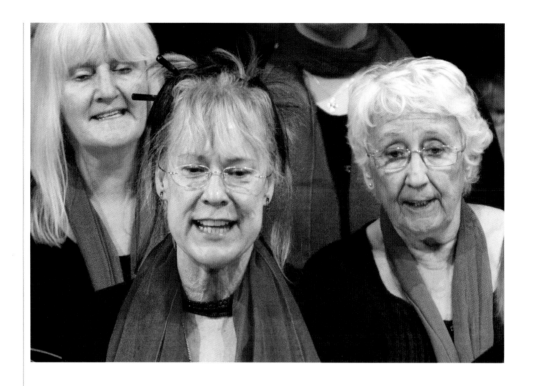

An individual case study of singing and lung disease

Jane Petto (centre) talks about her experience with singing and lung disease

"I'm ashamed to say that years of smoking took their toll on my health. I'd tried many times to quit but it was not until 1997 when I was told I had emphysema that I found the strength to stop. At this time a new women's choir 'Women in Harmony' was starting up in my home town of Tunbridge Wells. I joined as I thought a choir might give my lungs an extra work-out.

At the start of 2000 I started feeling ill and had a persistent cough. In August I was diagnosed with non-small cell lung cancer in my right lung. I was devastated. My mother had died of lung cancer in 1983. I didn't think there was any hope but my condition was operable and in October 2000 I had my right lung removed. Fortunately, I have been cancer free ever since.

Singing has been so good for my health. When I had my right lung removed I never imagined I would still be able to sing. At first I had only 40% lung capacity but two months after my operation I was singing again. Two years later because my lung muscles are strong from years of singing, it was found that my left lung was filling up the right side of my rib cage. My lung capacity had increased to 70%.

I now run a mixed choir called 'Folk in Harmony' in Crawley, Sussex. We sing all sorts – gospel, folk, do wop and songs from around the world. There're usually about 12 but we are always looking for new members. Several of the people in the choir had never sung before. I believe it's my job to build people's confidence and that it's everyone's birthright to sing. The choir is such a good way of getting you back on your feet again, which is what it did for me, and we have such a laugh. Singing has made such a difference to my life...especially after lung cancer. I'd recommend singing to everyone."

Based on Petto (2007)

Research evidence on singing and COPD

Innovative, cost-effective initiatives are needed to help people with COPD engage in physical and social activity to support independence and quality of life. There has been some research on the potential value of singing for people with COPD, but is an under-researched field which has only recently begun to attract attention.

Surveys have shown that choral singers believe that singing improves their breathing (Clift and Hancox, 2001, Clift, Hancox, Morrison et al. 2009) but comparison of lung function in professional singers versus wind and percussion players, failed to show significant differences in standard spirometric parameters (Clift, Hancox, Saricoff and Whitmore, 2008).

There is some evidence, however, that group singing may be beneficial for people with chronic respiratory disease by modifying breathing patterns, reducing breathlessness, and improving quality of life and social and psychological wellbeing. Engen (2005) recruited participants from a gerontology clinic and pulmonary rehabilitation clinic who had a diagnosis of emphysema. Twelve participants met in small groups twice a week for six weeks. None of the physical health and quality of life measures employed showed improvements over the six weeks of the study, but measures of breath control and voice intensity both improved significantly. In addition, breathing mode changed from being 'predominantly clavicular to 100% diaphragmatic that was maintained two weeks after the treatment sessions ended.'

Bonilha, Onofre, and Viera (2008) report a small randomised controlled trial assessing the impact of singing groups on lung function and quality of life among patients diagnosed with COPD. This study randomised 43 patients to a programme of singing or handcraft classes. Fifteen participants in each group completed 24 sessions. While the control group showed a decline in measures of maximal expiratory pressure, the group involved in singing showed a small improvement. Both groups showed increased quality of life scores with no significant difference, emphasising the benefits of group work.

A small trial examining the effects of singing lessons for patients with COPD has been completed at the Royal Brompton Hospital, London (Lord, Cave, Hume et al., 2010). Thirty-six COPD patients (mean FEV 37.2% predicted) were randomised to either 12 one-hour sessions of singing lessons over six weeks, or usual care. Following attrition 15 patients in the singing group were compared with 13 controls.

Significant improvements were found in levels of anxiety and self-assessed physical wellbeing in the singing group. Although no differences were found between the groups for 'single breath counting', incremental shuttle walking test (ISWT) scores or recovery time following ISWT, and surprisingly, breath-hold time increased more in the control group than the singing group. The study found therefore, that singing can be beneficial for the general wellbeing of people with COPD, but does not appear to have direct benefits on objective measures of lung function or physical performance.

However there was considerable value in what the group experience had for participants, and is demonstrated most clearly in the comments given during interviews. Eight patients were asked about the singing group and everyone was positive and no one reported any negative effects.

Positive physical effects described generally related to the breathing training which was a central aspect of the singing programme. The training encouraged feelings of control which many participants felt helped their breathing and eased their breathlessness.

"It has made my life easier; I would have liked this when I was first diagnosed."

"I increased my out-breath from 4 to 14 counts."

"I started breathing much better, from the stomach."

"The exercises, thinking about breathing and relaxing when I have (breathing) problems… this has been very useful."

Other positive physical effects described were an impact on lifestyle and functional ability:

"I have better posture now."

"Walking better, I go out more when it's not cold."

"Now things are less of a chore, housework is no longer a struggle."

Beneficial effects relating to general wellbeing were also very apparent:

"It was very enjoyable."

"It opened up a new lease of life."

"Emotionally… during singing it lifts you. I feel on top on the world. I also feel like that the day after. It makes COPD a lot easier to live with."

"Its uplifting to sing… this diagnosis is gloomy so the psychological effect of the group is good."

Practice

Guidance on setting up and running singing groups for COPD

The facilitator

The role of the facilitator is key in any musical group, and especially so in amateur choirs. The facilitator needs to be musically skilled but equally socially skilled and sensitive to the needs, circumstances and capacities of the people they are working with in a singing group. Musicians with experience of leading choirs, who are interested in working with people with COPD, may feel in need of training to understand the nature of the condition and the constraints it can place on people. A good way forward would be to contact organisations and projects with experience in this area to arrange a visit and explore possibilities for mentoring or training. Some ideas are given in the resource section of this guide.

The repertoire

A singing group for people with COPD is concerned first and foremost with meeting the psychological and social needs of the people involved. Therefore it is important for the range of music and songs to be wide to appeal to varied musical tastes in any group, and constructed and graded for progression. It is also important that the facilitator takes into account the breathing difficulties that participants might experience during singing. Particular emphasis needs to be placed on breathing and warm up exercises and on choosing and pacing songs in such a way that participants can comfortably take a breath as and when they need to. For example, songs that have worked well at the early stages of participation are: *Amazing Grace* and *We Are Sailing*.

Health and safety issues

Patients and carers would know not to attend if they were infectious with a chest infection for the sake of others, but it is as well to make this clear so that there is no misunderstanding. Patients carrying oxygen supplies are rightly wary of open fires or cigarette lighting or smoking. Obviously cigarette smoking shouldn't be taking place, but halls could perhaps be heated by open gas fires. Hall heating is very important, and the room should be up to temperature when the participants arrive. Entering a cold hall can be distressing for the patients and some halls are not able to maintain a warm temperature on the coldest days. Car parking should be close to the hall so that the distance walked is short and the patients are not out in the weather too long. Some may be in wheelchairs, but it is important those who aren't are provided with chairs.

Guidance on monitoring and evaluation

In setting up a new singing group for people with COPD it is important to consider the issue of monitoring and evaluation from the outset. Indeed if a group is funded by a statutory or voluntary body, some processes of evaluation and regular reports may be required. Gathering evidence on the process of outcomes of any project which aims to improve wellbeing and health is also essential to check whether the activity is having the desired effects.

Evaluation can be challenging and time-consuming to do well, and where possible the assistance of an external evaluator is ideal – not least because it gives some assurance of the independence and objectivity of the evidence gathered.

There are many approaches to evaluation, some simple and others more complex, and a wide range of techniques of information gathering and processing can be followed. Reference to previously published research described earlier in this guide can be useful in appreciating the range of approaches that have been adopted. For simplicity, however, here are three possibilities of increasing complexity:

Qualitative monitoring of process and outcomes

The simplest approach is to gather comments from participants on their experiences during the singing sessions and what they feel they have gained from their involvement. Simple questionnaires can be used for this purpose with some structured questions, but also space for people to write their own comments. The quotations given in the account of the Brighton and Hove Better Breathing singing groups above were gathered in just this way – by asking people to write open-ended accounts of their experiences in their singing groups.

Use of structured pre-validated questionnaires

A further step is to attempt to measure outcomes from participation in the singing groups using previously published questionnaires which are the result of a rigorous process of development and validation to show that they give meaningful results. A very commonly used questionnaire in research on COPD is the St George's Respiratory Questionnaire. This is readily available to use free of charge, but registration is required with Professor Paul Jones, who devised the questionnaire. A manual and scoring template is also available. This questionnaire takes about ten minutes for participants to complete, and so it makes very little demand on people. If participants are asked to complete them before the start of a singing group and then at intervals, it will be possible to see whether any improvements are taking place.

Controlled experiments on the effects of singing

The second approach to evaluation has the merit of attempting to measure change with a validated questionnaire. It has the obvious weakness however that the changes observed could have happened anyway or as a result of many other influences in people's lives in addition to being part of a choir. For this reason, some kind of 'control' group is often recommended in evaluations of any project to provide a point of comparison. In the ideal situation, such control groups would be established at the same time as the singing group and participants would be randomly assigned to the singing group and a control (either no intervention or some form of alternative activity). The evaluation undertaken by Lord et al. (2011) at the Royal Brompton and Harefield Hospital is a controlled study of this kind. Such studies are very expensive and time-consuming to set up and run.

Research ethics

If a 'singing for breathing' group is operating within the NHS, any evaluation or research project will require formal ethical approval through an NHS Local Ethics Committee. Where a group is operating in a community and participants refer themselves, and the group facilitator is keen to gather feedback, formal ethical approval would not be needed. It would still be important that information is gathered in accordance with sound ethical principles (e.g. informed consent and care over confidentiality and data protection). An important issue here is that of wishing to publish your results, which not only furthers the field, but also supports future funding applications. If you wish to publish in professional journals, they will require that the study has been through ethical approval.

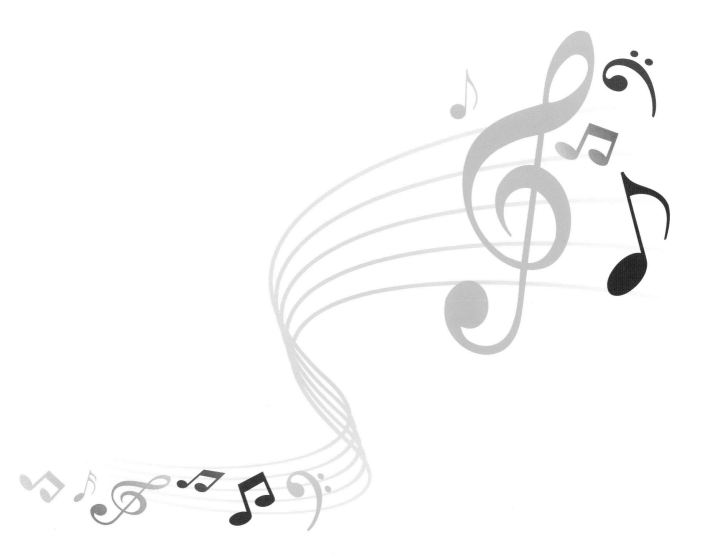

Sources of support and funding

There is increasing interest in the idea that singing can be beneficial for people with COPD and other breathing difficulties. Organisations and individuals with experience in this area are available to give help and support to anyone interesting in setting up new groups, and details can be found in the resources section in this guide.

Funding is a perennial challenge, although the costs involved in setting up and running a group are not very great. Funds are needed for the facilitators fee (and perhaps an accompanist or a system to play backing tracks), a venue and song sheets. Musicians should work with local Breathe Easy groups where they exist and respiratory and pulmonary rehabilitation services to discuss practical possibilities and sources of support. Local NHS health trusts and local commissioning consortia can be approached to explore sources of funding. For more ambitious projects, funders such as the Big Lottery and other charities with an interest in the arts could be approached.

The voluntary organisation Funding Buddies, is currently able to offer help with identifying sources of funding and a mentor scheme for bid-writing. They also offer a written toolkit (for Kent see **www.fundingbuddiesinkent.org.uk**).

With the increased introduction of personalised budgets for health and social care, this may also be a source of funding for singing for health groups, if participants, individually or collectively, choose to use some of their budget to pay for such an activity.

Resources

British Lung Foundation

One person in five in the UK is affected by lung disease. The British Lung Foundation (BLF) offer hope and support at every step, so that no one has to face it alone. They campaign for positive change in the nation's lung health and fund vital research into new treatments and cures. BLF are the UK's lung charity leading the fight against lung disease. www.blf.org.uk

Breathe Easy groups: The BLF's Breathe Easy support group network provides support and information for people living with a lung condition, and for those who look after them. You can meet others affected by lung disease at our free Breathe Easy support groups nationwide. Not only will you make new friends, you can get lots of information about lung disease at Breathe Easy meetings. Groups put on a varied programme of guest speakers and activities so you can learn to live with lung disease. Groups provide education and support for anyone affected by lung disease. www.blf.org.uk/BreatheEasy

Singing for breathing projects

Singing for Breathing (Folkestone): The 'Singing for Breathing' group in Folkestone was part of the wider East Kent 'Singing for Health' Network project. In June 2010, groups in the network came together for a performance event at The Granville Theatre, Ramsgate. For a short film based on this event see:
www.youtube.com/watch?v=MIsoii8pxO4

BetterBreathing singing groups (Brighton and Hove):
www.singforbetterhealth.co.uk
www.youtube.com/watch?v=GJ7RKpvu4LI

Singing for Breathing, Royal Brompton and Harefield Hospital (London): For a BBC report on this project, with COPD patients singing see: http://news.bbc.co.uk/1/hi/england/8189957.stm

Singing for Breathing, Nordoff Robbins London Centre:
Nordoff Robbins London Centre, 2 Lissenden Gardens, London NW5 1PQ
www.nordoff-robbins.org.uk

Music organisations for support and training

Natural Voice Practitioners Network: The Natural Voice Practitioners' Network is an organisation for Practitioners who share a common ethos and approach to voice work. NVPN believes that singing is everyone's birthright and they are committed to teaching styles that are accepting and inclusive of all, regardless of musical experience and ability. www.naturalvoice.net

Nordoff Robbins: Nordoff Robbins is a national charity that focuses on music therapy to support the lives of children and adults across the UK. The organisation also provides one-off or short programmes on developing musical skills and help with working with community groups. www.nordoff-robbins.org.uk

Sense of Sound: Sense of Sound's mission is to always be at the forefront of vocal education and to provide training, employment and promotional opportunities at the highest level in the creative industries for singers and songwriters across the UK and internationally. Sense of Sound delivers high-quality inclusive vocal training, develops and nurtures aspiring singers. www.senseofsound.org

Sound Sense: Sound Sense is a membership organisation that provides support to organisations and individuals who help people make music in their communities through leading music workshops and teaching. www.soundsense.org

References

Antonovsky, A. (1972) Breakdown: A needed fourth step in the conceptual armamentarium of modern medicine. Social Science and Medicine, 6, 537-544.

Antonovsky, A. (1987) Unravelling the Mystery of Health. How People Manage Stress and Stay Well. San Francisco, Jossey-Bass Inc.

Antonovsky, A. (1993) The structure and properties of the sense of coherence scale. Social Science and Medicine. 36, 6, 725-733.

Antonovsky, A. (1996) The salutogenic model as a theory to guide health promotion. Health Promotion International, 1996, 11, 1, 11-18.

Bengel, J. Strittmatter, R. and Willmann, H. (1999) What Keeps People Healthy? The Current State of Discussion and the Relevance of Antonovsky's Salutogenic Model of Health. Cologne: Federal Centre for Health Education.

British Lung Foundation (2007) Invisible lives: Chronic Obstructive Lung Disease (COPD) finding the missing millions, London: BLF.

Bonilha, A.G., Onofre, F., Vieira, L. M. et al. (2008) Effects of singing classes on pulmonary function and quality of life of COPD patients International Journal of COPD, 4, 1, 1-8.

Breathing Space (2010) Tune your lungs. Is singing really good for you? A pilot project in Folkestone is hoping to find out, Breathing Space, Spring 2010.

British Thoracic Society/British Lung Foundation (2002) Pulmonary Rehabilitation Survey, London: BTS/BLF.

Carstens, J. A. and Spangenberg, J. J. (1997) Major depression: A breakdown in sense of coherence? Psychological Reports, 80, 1211-1220.

Clift, S. and Hancox, G. (2001) The Perceived benefits of singing: findings from preliminary surveys with a university college choral society. Journal of the Royal Society for the Promotion of Health, 121, 4, 248-256.

Clift, S., Hancox, G., Morrison, I., Hess, B., Kreutz, G. and Stewart, D. (2009) What do singers say about the effects of choral singing on physical health? Findings from a survey of choristers in Australia, England and Germany, European Society for the Cognitive Sciences of Music (ESCOM) Conference, Jyvaskyla, Finland, 12-16 August, 2009.

Clift SM, Hancox G, Morrison I, Hess B, Kreutz G, Stewart D. (2010) Choral singing and psychological wellbeing: Quantitative and qualitative findings from English choirs in a cross-national survey. Journal of Applied Arts and Health, 1, 1, 19-34.

Clift, S. M., Hancox, G., Staricoff, R., Whitmore, C., with Morrison, I. and Raisbeck, M. (2008), Singing and Health: A Systematic Mapping and Review of Non-Clinical Studies, Canterbury: Canterbury Christ Church University. Available from: www.canterbury.ac.uk/research/centres/SDHR

Clift, S., Nicols, J., Raisbeck, M., Whitmore, C. and Morrison, I. (2011) Group singing, wellbeing and health: A systematic mapping of research evidence, The UNESCO Journal, 2, 1. Available from: www.abp.unimelb.edu.au/unesco/ejournal

Department of Health (2010a) Consultation on a Strategy for Services for Chronic Obstructive Pulmonary Disease (COPD) in England, London: Department of Health.

Department of Health (2010b) Equity and Excellence: Liberating the NHS, London: The Stationary Office.

Department of Health (2011) National Strategy to Transform Respiratory Disease Care, London: Department of Health.

Engen, R. (2005) The singer's breath: Implications for treatment of persons with emphysema. Journal of Music Therapy, 42, 20-48.

Fletcher, M., van der Molen, T., Salapatas, M. and Walsh, J. (2010) COPD Uncovered, London: Education for Health. Available from: www.educationforhealth.org/data/files/news/copd_report.pdf

Fraser, J., Page, S., and Skingley, Ann (2011) Drawing Breath: promoting meaning and self-management in COPD, British Journal of Community Nursing, 16, 2, 58-64.

Global Initiative for Chronic Obstructive Lung Disease, see: www.goldcopd.com

Halpin, D.M.G. (2003) Your Questions Answered: COPD, London: Churchill Livingstone.

Jones, P.W. (2009) Health status and the spiral of decline, COPD, 6, 59-63.

Lindstrom, B. and Eriksson, M. (2010) The Hitchhiker's Guide to Salutogenesis, Salutogenic Pathways to Health Promotion. Helsinki: IUHPE.

Lord V. M., Cave, P., Hume, V. et al. (2010) Singing teaching as a therapy for chronic respiratory disease – randomised controlled trial and qualitative evaluation, BMC Pulmonary Medicine, 10, 41, Available from: www.biomedcentral.com/1471-2466/10/41

National Institute for Health and Clinical Excellence (2010) Quick Reference Guide: Chronic Obstructive Pulmonary Disease, London: NIHCE.

Pavlicevic, M. and Ansdell, G. (2004) Community Music Therapy, London: Jessica Kingsley.

Petto, J. (2007) Jane Petto – Singer, Breathing Space, Spring 2007.

Thorax (2004) Diagnosing COPD, Thorax 2004, 59, i27-i38, Available from: www.thorax.bmj.com